Praise

'Dave's passion for supporting people who support kids is palpable. Creatively woven through *Challenging the Story* are stories that touch the heart and offer a transformative view of how we as adults can shift ourselves to be present to the children in our lives.'

— **Kim Barthel**, OTR, award-winning occupational therapist, best-selling author and multidisciplinary teacher on behaviour, neurobiology, trauma-sensitive practice, attachment, sensory processing, mental health, leadership and learning

'Empowering, practical, essential, memorable. Dave's book is a must-read for all who have or work with children. Weaving theoretical and practical wisdom, this book ultimately serves the highest health and happiness of present and future generations.'

— **Sonia Bestulic**, award-winning author, speaker, podcaster, speech pathologist and intuitive life coach

'*Challenging the Story* is a wonderful, engaging and captivating book that skilfully delves into the world of neurodivergent children. The ingenious use of characters not only brings the story to life but also serves as a powerful tool to educate readers about neurodiversity and how to support neurodivergent children in their learning environments – a must-read for educators, teachers, therapists and anyone involved in working with children.'

> — **Claire Joyce,** paediatric occupational therapist, director at Learn Through Play and author of the *How Does Your Body Feel?* boxset

Challenging the Story

A Surprisingly Simple Approach to **Supporting Children** with Challenging Behaviours

DAVID JEREB

ILLUSTRATED BY JULES FABER

Re think

First published in Great Britain in 2023
by Rethink Press (www.rethinkpress.com)

Contents

Introduction   1

   Challenging the Story companion guide   4

Prologue   7

1   Jenny's Class   9

2   The Beach Bean   13

3   Meeting Hoo   19

4   Challenging The Story   25

5   Misdirected Approach   31

6   Dysregulation   37

7   New Eyes   41

8   Antecedent   45

9   Unravelling The Layers   51

10   Research   57

11   Decoding The Triggers   63

12   Consequence   69

13   A Meaningful Solution   75

14   Parent–Teacher Interviews   81

15   The Playground   87

16   Behaviour Management Plan   91

17   Empowering With Responsibility   97

18   Staff Meeting   101

19   Goodbye, Mrs Hoo   107

Epilogue: The Wise Old Owl   **115**

Conclusion   **117**

MoveAbout Learning Pathways   120

MoveAbout Mentoring Program   120

MoveAbout Immersion Program   121

Acknowledgements   **123**

The Author   **127**

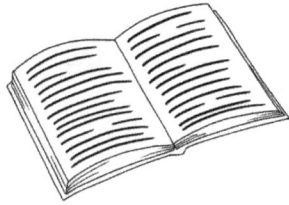

Introduction

In my career as a paediatric occupational therapist and mentor, I have been privileged to guide and support, and also learn from, countless children, families and fellow professionals. Through these experiences, I have often been astonished to discover how impactful it can be to shift our perspective on child behaviour. My wife Kathy and I co-founded MoveAbout Therapy Services, a paediatric occupational practice with three clinics in Australia, to support children and families to have meaningful lives and be their best versions of themselves. We do this by supporting the people who support the kids (our families, our team and our community). The insights I consider to be second nature in our work at MoveAbout Therapy Services have, at times, appeared revolutionary to those I mentor, and the families and educators we support. It is this realisation that inspired me to put pen to paper.

This book serves as an educational allegory, a blending of real-world experiences with strategies that have transformed the lives of many children and their families. It brings to life the principles that have shaped the ethos at MoveAbout – principles that have guided children with unique abilities and behaviours towards a path of successful learning and engagement. Each character, event and narrative woven into this book represents a child, a situation or a successful intervention I have encountered or implemented in my practice. All names and characters are fictional.

These tales are not mere stories, but reflections of the triumphs, struggles and enlightenments that my team and I have witnessed and been a part of.

They encapsulate our guiding principle – 'support the people who support the kids'.

While this book may appear to be about children and their behaviours, it's also about us, the adults in their lives. It's about parents, educators, health professionals and anyone else who plays a role in supporting children. It's about how we can shift our perspective and adapt our approach to transform not just the behaviours of the children we support but their entire life trajectory. It's also about how we ourselves can be transformed in this process.

If you've picked up this book, you are already taking an important step towards this transformation. I hope you find this story to be a practical guide in your interactions with children. I also hope the characters within this story stay in your mind and your heart, serving as models for you to reflect on as you face the challenges that each child's unique behaviours present. Thank you for joining me in this mission to seek to understand the child rather than focusing solely on the behaviour. My final hope is that this book challenges you, enlightens you and, ultimately, helps you to make a profound difference in the lives of the children you support.

Challenging the Story companion guide

To enrich your reading and learning experiences, I've designed a workbook specifically to help you internalise the key teachings of *Challenging the Story*. Each chapter is paired with three thought-provoking reflection questions, designed to help you relate the content to your daily experiences at work or home. This workbook is a must-have for individuals seeking a deeper understanding, and also serves as a lively conversation starter for team discussions or book club gatherings.

Before diving into the pages of this book, make sure you have this companion guide by your side. To get your free copy, simply visit the link or scan the QR code below.

www.moveabout.com.au/workbook

SCAN ME

Got your workbook? Fantastic! Now let's join Jenny on her journey and discover how we can challenge our initial interpretations of our kids' behaviours, guiding them towards a new and empowering narrative.

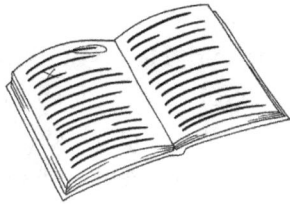

Prologue

Jenny sat on the couch with her laptop. Her air conditioner didn't seem to be touching the summer evening heat. She wiped her brow with her sleeve, hit save and shut down her computer. Her thoughts were spiralling.

As she looked up from her work, shifting her focus to the rerun of *Friends* that was playing on the TV, she thought to herself, *That's the lesson plan done, now I just have to work out how to get the kids to a place where I can teach them.* She closed the lid of the laptop and tuned back into the TV. Joey appeared on the screen and said 'How you doin'?'

'Not great, Joey, not great,' Jenny answered. Last week had been exhausting, and she'd wasted the whole weekend worrying about this week. She decided to switch off the TV too and head to bed. She needed all the energy she could gather for the working week.

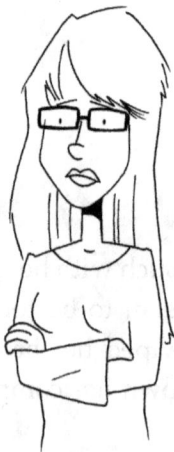

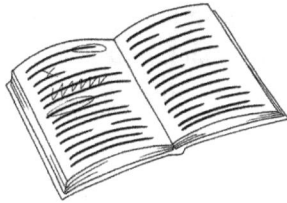

1
Jenny's Class

Jenny Jones was a first-grade teacher at Green Beach Public School. She'd been teaching for three years, but this year felt more difficult than even her first year. There seemed to be a lot more kids with challenging behaviours in her class, and a much greater range of abilities.

Three kids in particular took up a lot of her time: Jesse, Emma and Henry. Jesse, with his signature red headphones, was a sweet boy when he was with adults, but frequently reacted aggressively to the other kids. Emma was a nonspeaking autistic girl with black hair and a pale complexion, reminiscent of Snow White. She couldn't follow a lot of the curriculum and sometimes hit kids. Then there was Henry, the tallest in the class and a leader on the playground, who struggled with learning and often acted like the class clown, which made it hard for Jenny to teach.

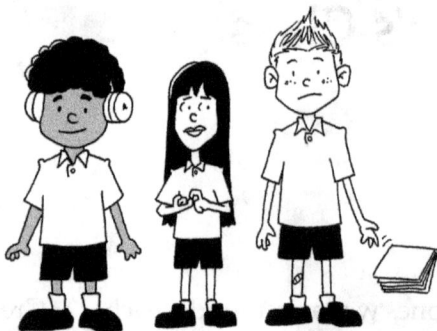

Jenny felt she was putting out so many fires each day that maybe she should have studied firefighting instead of teaching. Sometimes Jack, her classroom assistant, would turn to her panicked, looking for advice or direction. She'd race into action, often yelling and waving her hands – more like the person hoping to be rescued from the building than the firefighter.

Today was tough. In the morning, Emma looked like she wanted to play with John. She casually strolled up to him, reached out and hit him in the face, all with a smile on her face. John was in tears and Jenny had to race into action to soothe him while also trying to tell Emma her behaviour wasn't OK. When the class had eventually regrouped and found some order, the recess bell rang.

The day continued to flare into one fire after another. Jenny was feeling completely overwhelmed. This culminated in a chaotic session in the afternoon, when Jenny attempted to have the class catch up on the literacy lesson they'd missed in the morning's commotion. She decided to have the students read aloud as a group. When it was Henry's turn to read, he took the book, seemed to freeze for a second, and then said 'Blah, blah, blah' in a silly voice, making the whole class laugh. Exasperated, Jenny sent Henry to the principal's office.

She had lost the room.

To top it off, in all the turmoil Jesse bit George on the shoulder. The school day could not end soon enough.

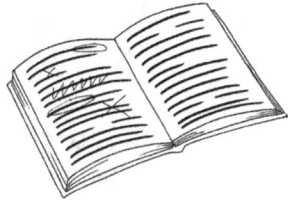

2
The Beach Bean

Jenny was looking forward to this afternoon. She was catching up with her co-worker and best friend, Allie – also a teacher at Green Beach Public – for a cuppa by the beach. Allie had been teaching for eight years now, with five of those years in Green Beach.

Jenny squinted in the afternoon glare as she got out of her car. She allowed her eyes to adjust for a second as she tuned into the sight of the ocean and the sound of the waves. The Beach Bean, with its blue-and-white weathered wood panel walls and plastic furniture, was one of her favourite places to unwind.

They had driven separately, and when Jenny arrived Allie had already secured a table outside and had even ordered for her. 'Skinny white chocolate mocha.' Allie pointed to the tasty beverage that was waiting on the table.

Jenny greeted Allie with a pressed smile, sat down and took a big gulp of her mocha. 'Mmm, I needed that.'

'How was your day?' Allie asked.

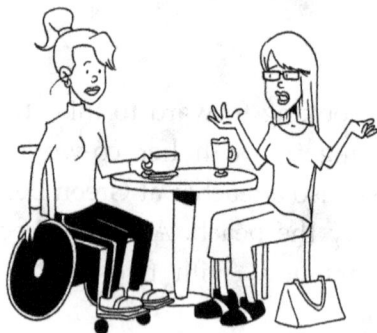

That question was all it took for tears to well up in Jenny's eyes. 'I don't know that I'm cut out for teaching anymore,' she responded.

'What happened?' enquired Allie with a compassionate smile.

Jenny took a breath and unloaded her day, mentioning the incident at reading time. She also spoke about how she had thought Emma was becoming more social, until she whacked John in the face. 'Is it just me or are the classes getting harder and harder?'

'Wow, that is a big day!' Allie exclaimed. 'Sounds like enough to drive you to drink. Drink something chocolatey and caffeinated, I mean,' she said, attempting to lighten the mood.

'Every day feels like a big day.' Jenny sighed. 'I just don't know what I can do to help all these kids. I've tried stickers and reward charts, praise and time outs. None of it seems to be making a difference. Oh Allie, what am I going to do?'

Allie gave a soft smile. She took a second, connecting with Jenny eye to eye, soul to soul. 'Jenny, honey, you don't need a what, you need a who – someone who has been through it all before. Someone with knowledge and experience.'

'OK, I'm listening.' Jenny leaned in a little.

Allie paused for a second longer, and then, with a cheeky smile, she said, 'Jenny, you need to talk to Hoo!'

'I need to talk to who?'

'That's right!'

'What's right?'

'You need to talk to Hoo.'

'I don't know, that's what I'm asking you. Who do I need to talk to?'

'You need to talk to Hoo – Mrs Hoo, the wise old owl. Hoooo,' Allie exclaimed in her best owl impression.

'Who's Mrs Hoo?' Jenny questioned, more confused than ever.

'She's a legend in the school district. She seems to be able to connect with any kid and help them improve how they behave and engage in class. She's technically retired, but she's been doing some casual teaching. Principal Davies said she's covering Tom Reed's class while he's travelling for the next few months.'

'Wow, she does sound like someone I'd like to talk to,' Jenny responded with intrigue and a hint of hope.

'I have her number, I'll send her a message and let her know you could use a hand. I'm sure she'd be glad to help.'

'That would be amazing!' Jenny felt a sense of relief already.

Allie typed the text message there and then. She hit send and the sound triggered a mixture of feelings for Jenny. First, she quickly inhaled with anticipation, and then she gave a long breath out, feeling a small sense of relief.

They moved on to talk about other things beyond work, and before they knew it the sun was beginning to set and it was time to say goodbye. 'See you tomorrow, Jen,' Allie said. 'I'll let you know when I hear back from Mrs Hoo.'

'Whooooo?' questioned Jenny with a smirk. 'Thanks Allie, see you tomorrow.' They hugged and headed off in different directions.

Later that night, Allie texted Jenny to say that Mrs Hoo would be happy to speak with her and that she should catch her in the staffroom on Monday. Jenny thanked her again, switched her phone to silent and tried to get to sleep early. It took her a long time to fall asleep as she tried to imagine what Mrs Hoo could possibly tell her that could make her life easier.

'Jenny, honey, you don't need a what, you need a who – someone who has been through it all before. Someone with knowledge and experience.'

REFLECTION POINT

When you face a problem or challenge, it can be helpful to seek out someone who's been through a similar situation. They can provide invaluable insights based on their experiences. Remember, there's always someone willing to lend a hand, particularly to those who are in the service of supporting children. The first step is often the hardest – you have to ask for help. Don't be afraid to do so; it's a sign of strength and wisdom to recognise when you need it, and to have the courage to ask.

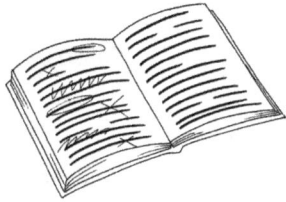

3

Meeting Hoo

Jenny arrived at work early on Monday, hoping that she would run into Mrs Hoo before the day started, but she didn't see her before the morning bell. Jenny was on playground duty at recess so she missed her on that break too. When the lunch bell rang, she led her class out into the playground and hurried to the staffroom.

When she arrived, she saw a woman she had never met before sitting on the soft blue couch, reading some paperwork with the school letterhead. She had dark hair, streaked with silver, and wore a gold blouse and stylish jade glasses. Mrs Hoo's face was lined with wrinkles, which seemed to accentuate her kind smile. Her eyes sparkled with intelligence and she gave the impression of having a deep understanding of children. There was a sense of firmness and no-nonsense about her, as if she had seen it all before and knew exactly what needed to be done.

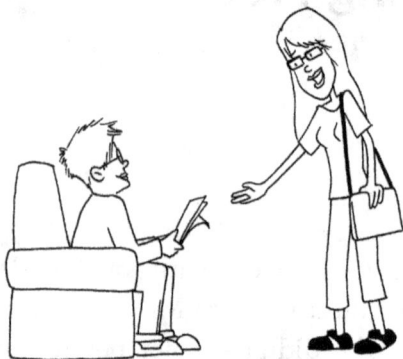

'Excuse me, are you Mrs Hoo?' Jenny asked.

Mrs Hoo looked up from her papers and replied in a friendly tone, 'Yes, that's me. You must be Jenny, am I right?'

'Yes,' replied Jenny. 'Would you mind if I asked you a few questions? People say you're pretty wise.'

Mrs Hoo chuckled. 'I'm glad you stopped before the old and owl part,' she said with a playful wink. 'Why don't we go somewhere quieter? I expect this place will get busy soon.'

Jenny agreed, and they gathered their lunches and headed to Jenny's classroom.

Jenny had only one adult-sized chair so they both sat on the kids' chairs at one of the children's desks. The only interesting features of the cream-coloured desk were a smiley face drawn in pencil on the corner, a dusting of eraser shavings and a sticky streak of glue that had collected a variety of dust, fluff and dirt. The walls were busy with letters and numbers, and displayed a plethora of children's artwork.

Jenny sat down nervously, unsure where to start. Mrs Hoo had been recommended by Allie as a wise and experienced teacher who could offer some guidance, and now here she was sitting across from Jenny, ready to be asked for help. Jenny took a deep breath and began to explain the challenges she had been facing in her classroom, hoping Mrs Hoo could offer some insights and strategies to help her better support her students.

'The day I met with Allie and she messaged you, that was a tough day,' she said. Her pace quickened as she relived the emotional roller coaster of the day. 'I had Emma smiling as she attacked John by hitting him in the face, and Henry acting like the class clown during reading time, making everyone laugh, which seemed to set off Jesse who then bit George on the shoulder. The class spiralled into total chaos. It feels like I'm putting out fires all day.'

Mrs Hoo listened attentively then nodded. 'It sounds like a challenging day, indeed,' she said.

'I'm sorry,' Jenny replied. 'My thoughts are pouring out all jumbled. You must be wondering what you've gotten yourself into.'

'Not at all,' Mrs Hoo responded warmly. 'I am wondering something though: why are you so hard on yourself? Jenny, I need to tell you, your class is a challenging mix of kids. You can't be expected to figure this out alone, and I'm happy to help. One thing is clear – you care deeply for those kids and you are determined to find some answers to help them.'

Mrs Hoo's words were soothing to Jenny. They reminded her of the way her grandmother spoke to her when she'd grazed her knee at the park or had made a spelling mistake on her homework as a child.

'Your class is a challenging mix of kids. You can't be expected to figure this out alone, and I'm happy to help.'

REFLECTION POINT

Navigating the challenges of interacting with and understanding a diverse group of children is no mean feat, be it as an educator, parent or caregiver. Jenny's encounter with Mrs Hoo sheds light on the importance of seeking guidance and collaboration in the face of adversity. It's a testament to the reality that one doesn't always have to have all the answers, but rather the willingness to seek them.

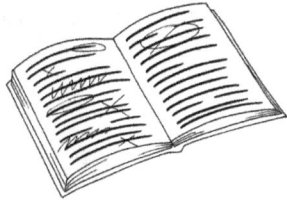

4

Challenging The Story

'Let me tell you a story,' Mrs Hoo continued. 'In my past life, before I retired…' She raised an eyebrow and gave a wry smile at her inability to commit to the concept of retirement. She loved what she did too much.

'In my past life, I used to support teachers like you across the whole district. I was frequently called in because a child was attacking other kids.' She used finger quotes to accentuate the word 'attacking'.

'Tell me, Jenny, do you think this is a subjective or objective description of what was happening?'

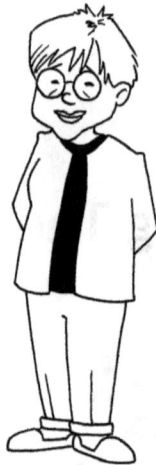

Jenny paused. 'That seems like a trick question. Objective means the facts of what happened, whereas subjective means our opinion or interpretation, right?' Mrs Hoo nodded.

'I see this all the time in our class,' Jenny continued. 'So, it feels objective. We see, with our own eyes, the child going up and whacking another kid.' She looked at Mrs Hoo, trying to read her expression. 'I think you're going to tell me otherwise.'

'Very perceptive, Jenny. I do believe it's subjective and gives the sense that the child is being intentionally aggressive when we don't really know that. Saying it's aggressive is saying that they're doing it on purpose, which is our opinion, since we can't jump into the child's mind. How could we phrase it more objectively?'

'Hitting the other child?' Jenny suggested.

'Closer, but it still gives a sense of judgement. How about, "Moving their hand in the direction of the other child's face"?' She paused to let this sink in.

Jenny looked unconvinced. This seemed a step too far. 'Surely we know that it's hitting? Why isn't that objective?'

'Hmm,' Mrs Hoo responded, 'sometimes when we think we know the story, we need to pause, look a little more closely and see if there is a second story of the behaviour that we have missed.' She held Jenny's gaze. 'When I was called in to these classes, I'd often come to observe the child doing this behaviour, and I would see one of three possible things. In the first scenario, the child would be playing with toys, really focusing on a toy. Another child would come along and reach for one of their toys, potentially brushing past them with a light touch. The first child would react defensively as they were caught off guard; they were surprised, felt threatened and may also have disliked the light touch or the sound. In this case, it's our job as adults to better support and facilitate these interactions.

'When we see it happening, we can move into a coaching mode and suggest to the other child they approach from the front, so the first child can see them coming. We can also use a warm voice to help the first child see that the other child is friendly and wants to play, and we can possibly even facilitate parallel play where they both have similar toys.'

'Ah, I can see that you've redefined the behaviour as defensive rather than aggressive, and that changes the whole way we would approach handling it. This child reminds me of Jesse.'

'Yes, he came to my mind too. The first story you had of his behaviour was that he was being aggressive by biting the other child, but if we look more closely, we see that there may be a second story of a child who is not aggressive but defensive and responding to protect himself. For Jesse, it seems like the sound may have set him off. This gives you the opportunity, which is in fact also a necessity, to use different strategies to help him be successful in your class and keep him and others safe.'

Jenny nodded, chewing on her bottom lip as she made mental notes. *Always start with the objective behaviour,* she thought, *and remove personal feelings from the equation.* She repeated these words silently, underlining them in her mind.

> '*Sometimes when we think we know the story, we need to pause, look a little more closely and see if there is a second story of the behaviour that we have missed.*'

REFLECTION POINT

Shifting from a subjective to an objective perspective is crucial when understanding and managing behaviour. By stepping back and looking at behaviour objectively, we gain deeper insights into its underlying drivers. This shift allows us to explore alternative interpretations and consider the 'second story' behind a child's actions. Embracing objectivity opens new avenues for effective strategies, empathy and support. Behaviour is complex and influenced by various factors, and adopting an objective lens leads to better outcomes for both the child and the adults supporting them.

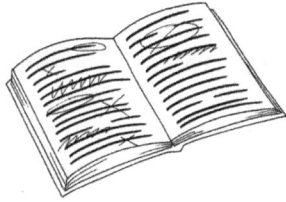

5

Misdirected Approach

Mrs Hoo continued, 'The next scenario involves a type of child that reminds me of your student Emma. Would you like to hear about that child?'

Jenny leaned forward, her eyes wide with eagerness. 'Yes, definitely!' she exclaimed. 'Just when I think we're making progress, we hit a setback. I'm interested to understand more about this.'

'You mentioned Emma is autistic, is that correct?'

'Yes, that's right.'

'I've worked with many autistic kids. Eye contact tends to be challenging for them, which means they may miss the social cues and nonspeaking aspects of communication.'

'That sounds like Emma,' Jenny reflected out loud. 'Although, she does seem to be using it more often these days and is happy about engaging with others, which I think is a positive sign.'

'It certainly is,' Mrs Hoo answered, validating Jenny, appreciating the fact that Jenny was truly immersed in the discussion and learning.

'Sometimes the child also has poor motor planning, meaning they are not good at planning their movements to meet the demands of the situation. Now, if you'll forgive me going off on a tangent, my five-month-old grandson will sit in my lap and bat my face with his hands. It's gorgeous. I'll pretend to gobble his hands. I could do it all day.

'To return to Emma, it's not so gorgeous to others when the child is older and bigger and batting at their face, but the intention may be the same. The child may be trying to engage the other child. Her reach towards them is an approach behaviour, an overture to initiate play; however, it is certainly not perceived that way by the other child, or by the adults for that matter.'

Jenny sat silently, letting this all soak in. Her mind was officially blown. It made so much sense.

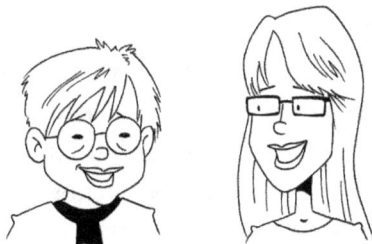

'With Emma,' Mrs Hoo continued, 'you've worked hard to support her to move from being disconnected and in her own world to feeling safe and allowing others into her world, and also to being interested in others and their worlds. The fact that she's now approaching and initiating interactions with other kids is a sign of amazing progress. That doesn't mean you do nothing, but what you need to do is also different from an aggressive behaviour.

'Like with the defensive child, you need to facilitate interactions, to coach and provide support and guidance. As you see her approach, you may say, "Emma, it looks like you want to play with John. You can wave or say play." If you arrive late, you could say, "Uh-oh, John seemed surprised when you reached for his face. You could touch his arm," and then show her with your own hand.

'To John, you could say, "Whoops, Emma was reaching out to play, but it looks like she surprised you. She doesn't have a lot of words; can she touch your arm or hands when she wants to ask to play?"

'John still gets to choose whether this is OK or not but, by doing this, you're starting to help everyone understand what's happening and coach them towards a more positive interaction. Emma is learning through this process, and John now has more context for why Emma touched his face.'

'Wow!' exclaimed Jenny. 'That makes so much sense and feels so much better. I like that story of Emma's behaviour much more than the confusing one I had before. It stressed me out because there seemed to be such a mismatch between the behaviour and her facial expression. I found that almost harder than when a child is angry.'

'The child may be trying to engage the other child. Her reach towards them is an approach behaviour, an overture to initiate play; however, it is certainly not perceived that way by the other child, or by the adults.'

REFLECTION POINT

Understanding behaviour, especially in children who have difficulty engaging and relating, including those with autism, requires a deeper dive into their intentions, emotions and actions. A behaviour that might seem aggressive or out of place to an outsider may be an innocent and positive gesture from the child's perspective. Adopting an empathetic and informed approach to these behaviours can not only change our perspective but also significantly enhance our ability to guide and support these children.

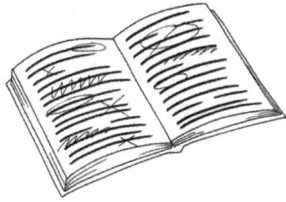

6
Dysregulation

'Nice segue to the third example I want to share.' Mrs Hoo took control again. 'The third type of child does appear to be approaching the other child to hit them. They might look angry or upset. In this scenario it is more challenging to view their actions with positive regard and to work out the plot of that new story. It often relates to something that's just happened (and maybe we missed it), the child's profile or their previous experiences with this child or others, or even previous traumatic experiences.

'Regardless of why they are doing it, they are almost always dysregulated when they do it. When someone is dysregulated, they find it difficult to access their executive functions; that is, their thinking and reasoning brain and their language. This means that strategies requiring them to remember, think ahead or problem-solve are off the table. It also means they won't be able to process a lot of language at that time.'

'So that's why, no matter how well the child can say the rules or the consequences, sometimes they still do things they shouldn't when they're upset.'

'Exactly!'

As Mrs Hoo said the word 'exactly', the bell rang. It was time for them to return to their classes.

They stood up to leave. 'I hope that feels helpful,' Mrs Hoo said. 'Why don't you let that all percolate, and we can catch up again in a few days. How about we get together after school on Thursday at that place down by the beach?'

'The Beach Bean. Yes, that sounds fantastic,' Jenny confirmed. 'Thank you so much. That was unbelievably helpful. I feel like I will be looking at my kids with fresh eyes, and maybe I can help them write a new story of their behaviour.'

'I'm glad to hear it,' replied Mrs Hoo. 'Now, I better go before the principal makes me follow through on my retirement.' She mocked concern, eyes wide, and then gave a cheeky wink. They shared a warm smile and Mrs Hoo turned and left the classroom.

As the kids began to line up outside the room, Jenny felt a combination of hope and excitement as she thought about this huge boost of knowledge she'd just received and how she was now going to be better able to help the kids in her class.

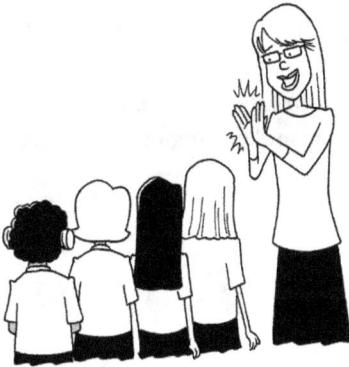

'When someone is dysregulated, they find it difficult to access their executive functions; that is, their thinking and reasoning brain and their language.'

REFLECTION POINT

Understanding the intricacies of dysregulation is paramount for educators, caregivers and anyone who interacts with children. When children are dysregulated, they might behave in ways that can seem bewildering or out of character; however, it's not born out of a desire to be defiant, but is instead a result of their emotional state compromising their cognitive capacities. The profound revelation that children, during these heightened emotional times, might not be accessing their thinking and reasoning brain prompts us to shift our perspective. Rather than viewing them as intentionally disruptive, we're encouraged to see them as individuals in need of support. Rather than expecting rational behaviour, the response to such children should, ideally, be infused with patience, empathy and strategies tailored to their current emotional state.

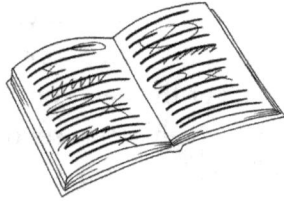

7
New Eyes

Jenny met with Jack the next day. She shared what Mrs Hoo had taught her about viewing the children's actions objectively. Although Jack understood the concept, he was initially sceptical. 'That sounds interesting,' he said, 'but do you think it'll make a difference?'

'Honestly, Jack, I do,' Jenny replied. 'I can't explain it quite like Mrs Hoo, but can we give it a go?'

'Sure we can,' said Jack. He was a trusting ally to Jenny and had such compassion for the kids in their class. Jenny couldn't ask for a more committed teammate. 'I'm happy to give it a go.'

Over the next couple of days, Jenny felt like she'd been given a new set of eyes. When things happened in her classroom, she could now see the behaviours more objectively, which meant her responses were much more effective.

When Jesse was playing with the train set, Jenny made sure to keep an eye out. When another child approached, Jesse shouted 'No!' Jenny raced over.

'Uh-oh, Rosie, you surprised Jesse.' She took a deep breath. 'Hey, Jesse, I think Rosie thinks your game is cool. Rosie, how about we set you up with some trains and tracks here?' Jesse's shoulders relaxed, and he took a breath that matched Jenny's.

When Emma approached George and reached out with her hand, Jenny tried to help her use a more engaging gesture. She also tried to model this gesture, initiating her own interactions with Emma by getting in front of her, reaching her hands forward and saying 'Play?'

When Jesse covered his ears and moved away from the group during music, Jack went over to ask him to return, but decided to first check in with him. 'Are you OK, mate?'

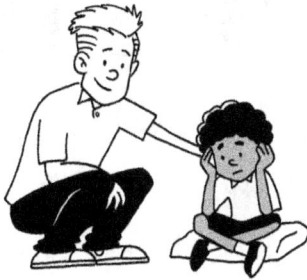

'It's too loud over there,' Jesse replied defensively. He was worried that Jack was going to make him rejoin the group. Instead, Jack gave him a nod. 'Yeah, it is pretty loud isn't it.' He realised that Jesse wasn't leaving the group to misbehave, he was sensitive to the sound of the musical instruments.

Jack put a few instruments in front of Jesse and then sat next to him. He didn't talk about them, he just placed them down. After a few minutes, Jesse picked up the drum. He smiled as he beat it in time with the music. It seemed he wasn't nearly as sensitive to the noise when he controlled the instrument. Jack was pleased that Jesse was able to be part of the activity, and even play some instruments, albeit from a bit of a distance.

Jenny looked at Jack and gave him a thumbs up. She was so excited about the progress she and their class had made. She couldn't wait to share the stories with Mrs Hoo.

She could now see the behaviours more objectively, which meant her responses were much more effective.

REFLECTION POINT

The power of objective observation and intervention cannot be underestimated. Our ability to observe and understand behaviours improves with deliberate practice. When we step back and view behaviours without subjective judgement, we gain a clearer understanding of what is truly happening. By honing our observational skills, we can identify the underlying reasons behind behaviours and respond in ways that support and engage children effectively. When we look at the 'what' objectively, considering 'how' it is done, it helps us to begin to understand 'why' it is happening. Then a new story unfolds and provides an opportunity to support the child proactively rather than reacting as we try to deal with the behaviour in the moment.

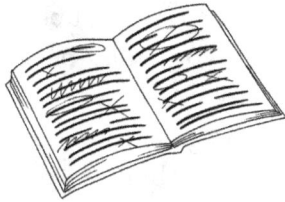

8
Antecedent

On Thursday afternoon, Jenny hurried to The Beach Bean. The overcast sky had no impact on her bright spirit. The Beach Bean was packed already with the after-school rush. Jenny looked around for a table. Surprisingly, when she walked to the balcony Mrs Hoo was waiting for her there.

'Good afternoon, Jenny.' Mrs Hoo called her over, the corners of her vibrant emerald eyes crinkling in a warm welcome. She gestured for Jenny to join her.

Jenny was bubbling with excitement. 'Hi, Mrs Hoo, you won't believe everything that's happened in my class since we spoke!' She burst into a list of all the great things that had happened, now that she had the ability to better understand the behaviours her kids were displaying. She told Mrs Hoo all about her interactions with Emma and Jesse, and the music class where Jack also supported Jesse.

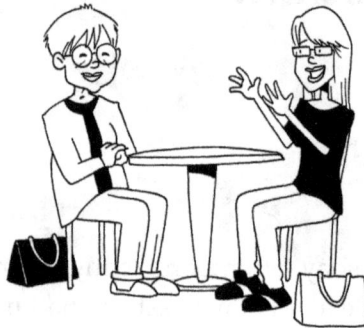

She finished recapping the successes of the week and how she, Jack and the class were changing so quickly. At the end she smiled and said, 'Jack suggested we should get bracelets made up that say "WWHD?"'

'WWHD?' Mrs Hoo queried.

'What would Hoo do?' Jenny explained with a giggle.

Mrs Hoo raised her eyebrows and then gave an understanding smile and nod of acknowledgement.

Then Jenny had a thought. 'I'm so sorry. I just started jabbering and forgot that we should order our drinks. This place is so busy of an afternoon, it can take a while.'

As if by magic, the waiter appeared, but he wasn't there to take their orders. 'Green tea and a skinny white chocolate mocha.' He placed the drinks in front of the ladies.

'Thanks,' Jenny said to the waiter. She turned to Mrs Hoo. 'How did you know my order?'

'I do my research' – Mrs Hoo gave a small giggle, punctuated with a wink – 'and so should you. You mentioned you are dealing a lot better with the behaviours in your class now you are perceiving them more objectively, but are you preventing them yet?'

'Somewhat,' Jenny said. 'Although, mostly they're still happening; we're just dealing with them a bit better.'

'That's a good start. The next step is seeing if we can prevent them from happening. Wouldn't that be better for the kids, and for you?'

'It sure would,' Jenny exclaimed, 'but how do we do that? We've had lots of behaviour management plans but, as you mentioned, the kids don't have the executive functions – the higher-level thinking – to use those strategies or understand the consequences when they're not regulated, and they're almost never regulated when the behaviours happen. That's half the reason they happen.'

Mrs Hoo gave an understanding smile. 'You have listened and learnt a lot from our last conversation, and you're right. Often they are not regulated when the behaviours occur, and so they can't make a different choice' – she paused – 'on their own; but hopefully you *are* regulated.'

Jenny's eyes shifted up and to the left as she absorbed what she'd just heard. 'You're right,' she said. 'I'm the adult. It's up to me to help my kids. I have been trying. I keep an eye out for Jesse and Emma during free time because that's usually when things happen, but often they just seem to happen without warning.'

'Perhaps,' Mrs Hoo responded, 'or perhaps you just haven't identified the antecedent.'

'Ah, yes. The antecedent,' Jenny said. 'I see where you're going here. You're referring to the ABCs of behaviour management. We learnt about them at uni, and we need to list them on the Behaviour

Management Form. Last time you helped me identify the behaviour… objectively.' She emphasised the word 'objectively'. 'That's the B. Now I need to get better at understanding the antecedent. The thing that typically comes before the behaviour.'

'Wow, I'm not sure you need me. Maybe you just need a good pen, a piece of paper and a skinny white chocolate mocha!'

'No, I do need you,' Jenny responded emphatically. 'I've filled out those sheets but I don't really know the antecedent for most of the behaviours. They just seem to happen.'

> *'Now I need to get better at understanding the antecedent. The thing that typically comes before the behaviour.'*

REFLECTION POINT

Understanding antecedents is key to addressing challenging behaviours. By examining the context and events leading up to the behaviour, we gain valuable insights into the underlying causes. Antecedents go beyond immediate triggers and encompass the broader context, including experiences, routines and environment. Identifying and understanding antecedents allows us to proactively intervene and create supportive conditions that prevent behaviours. It helps us move from a focus on the 'what' of the behaviour to the 'why' of the behaviour. It allows us to be more proactive in our approach to supporting children and developing a new story that has the child, rather than the behaviour, at the centre.

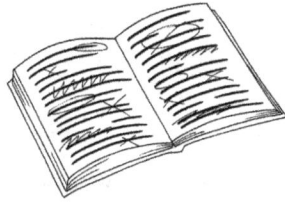

9
Unravelling The Layers

'Jenny, these behaviours may just seem to happen; however, in your stories of how you and Jack have begun to support your class by viewing their behaviour objectively, you've provided several examples of antecedents. You saw that Emma wanted to play with others. That's an antecedent for her behaviour that you're trying to understand. Jack discovered that Jesse moved away because he was sensitive to the sound in your music lesson. That means loud sounds are an antecedent that can lead to Jesse leaving the group. This also provides you with some important information about his underlying capacities.

'In terms of your behaviour management plans, the problem may be that you've been looking for the antecedent rather than the antecedents.' She now accentuated the 's'. 'Some behaviours are complex and, consequently, so are the reasons behind them and the necessary responses.

'Finally, regulation and behaviour don't happen in a vacuum. They occur in a context and across time. The antecedent may not occur right before the behaviour, but at some point during the entire lead-up. It could start with how breakfast and getting out of the house went, or even with how the child slept the night before.'

'Wow, that makes so much sense. How can I ever know all that?'

'You can't. You can't know all of that, but if you understand even some of that, you will be much better off, and, more importantly, so will the kids.

'Here's what you're going to do…' She paused, checking that Jenny was ready. Jenny sat up straight, ready to receive her homework. 'I think you should identify one objective behaviour for each of the kids you spoke to me about, and then track when each behaviour happens across the day. Whenever you have a chance, go back and jot down what happened in the lead-up. Include what happened for the child, but also what activities they were doing and what was going on in the environment.'

'Consider it done,' Jenny declared with a look of conviction. 'I'll get Jack to help me.'

'Great idea. One more thing: see if their parents would be happy to share a bit more information about how their child's day has started, and even their sleep the night before. Anything they think might be relevant. When the child has difficulty communicating, the adults need to be excellent at communicating,' Mrs Hoo finished.

Jenny felt electrified with new ideas and strategies. 'We have a communication book we use. I'll give those parents a call and chat to them about adding a bit more detail and about why it's helpful. I should probably communicate the same kind of information to them when I send the communication book home.'

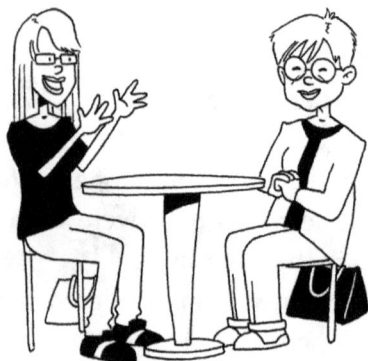

'Yes, that would be a good idea, but be mindful that you're not just being negative. Parents hear the negatives a lot. Give them the information that helps them support their child, but also let them know you're an ally and that you see the beauty in their child.'

Jenny absorbed this important message in silence, giving a nod of acknowledgement.

They had finished their drinks and also their lesson. 'Well, I think that's enough homework for today,' Mrs Hoo said. 'Why don't you get started on that and we can meet back here in a week?'

'OK,' said Jenny. 'I'll work with Jack to identify our key goal behaviours for each child, and we'll start collecting the data. I'll chat to their parents about using their communication books more effectively.'

They walked to the counter and paid for their drinks. Jenny thanked Mrs Hoo one more time and they said goodbye. Jenny walked to her car, her mind swirling with thoughts and plans.

'In terms of your behaviour management plans, the problem may be that you've been looking for the antecedent rather than the antecedents.' She now accentuated the 's'.

REFLECTION POINT

Every individual's behaviour is influenced by a myriad of factors, and often exists in layers of complexity. Recognising there may not be a singular antecedent, but rather a series of antecedents that interact and accumulate, is crucial in understanding and supporting positive behaviour change. By seeking deeper insights into a child's day, environment and experiences, we can begin to uncover these intricate layers. This broader perspective emphasises the importance of consistent communication among all caregivers and advocates in the child's life. True understanding and effective support come not from isolating individual triggers but from weaving together the multiple threads that influence behaviour. Through this holistic approach, we position ourselves not just as observers, but as allies in the child's story.

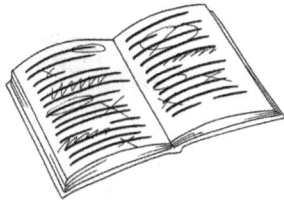

10
Research

Jenny discussed the plan with Jack and he was on board with helping to create the sheet and collect the information. They created a data collection sheet that included their session plan for the day, which focused on five key points – the behaviour, its timing, the ongoing activity, what happened before the behaviour and what happened after the behaviour – along with any general notes for context. This straightforward approach gave them a holistic view of each incident to identify patterns and triggers.

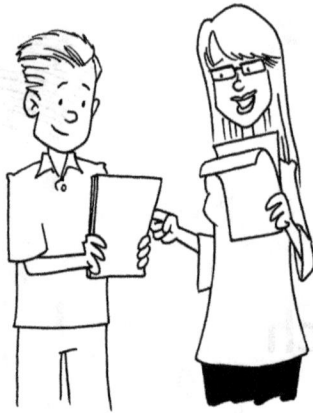

The next day, they started collecting data on the goal behaviours. With the sheet they'd created, the process was relatively easy. Initially, amid the chaos of the classroom, they occasionally forgot to use the sheet, but they quickly adapted and soon it became second nature. By lunchtime on the second day, they were in a groove and collecting data like academic researchers.

As they became more observant of the kids, they realised they were becoming better able to identify when a child's behaviour was escalating, and to identify cues that could help them see when the child was beginning to dysregulate. For instance, Jenny noticed that Jesse's shoulders would tense up and his smile would turn into an uncomfortable grimace. This often occurred when the room became louder or more chaotic during free time, music time and transitions between activities. Previously, she had just assumed he was smiling, but now she could tell the difference between a genuine, relaxed smile and a retracted, strained smile.

Jack noticed something similar with Emma. While Jenny had spoken to Mrs Hoo about the times when Emma was smiling and reaching for other kids, Jack also noticed that there were times when Emma's body language was different. She would look disorganised, unfocused and begin to grind her teeth. Sometimes she also pushed or hit the other students in this state. They realised that this behaviour wasn't aggressive, but neither was it a calm approach for connection. It was defensive. She was overwhelmed and needed some space. They could now tell the difference, and began to see this in the lead-up to situations.

With Henry, they noticed that his behaviour always happened during literacy lessons, particularly when he was asked to read or talk in front of the class. As soon as someone suggested the children would be expected to read, Henry became fidgety and his breathing became short and shallow, almost as if he was holding his breath. He seemed to hold it together unless the attention was on him. When he became the focus during the reading activity, he inevitably displayed some kind of behaviour that led to him getting into trouble and being removed from the activity.

By identifying the antecedents of these behaviours, they understood the children better and read their cues so they could help them before the challenging behaviour occurred.

Jenny spoke on the phone to Emma's and Henry's mothers and Jesse's father about adding more detail in the communication book, including how the morning had gone and any other information that might be relevant and impacting the child's behaviour, such as how they slept the night before. She explained why this would be helpful. She also offered to provide more information to the families. They were all receptive and more than willing to provide more information themselves, particularly if it could help their child.

Henry's mother spoke quietly and cautiously as she told Jenny he had always gotten into trouble for 'mucking up in class' but she knew he was a smart kid. She also mentioned reading had always been hard for Henry. She took a breath before sharing that it had been hard for her as a child too. Jenny listened intently. Henry's mother graciously thanked Jenny for seeing that his clowning around was more than just 'naughty behaviour'. Jenny could sense that Henry's mother was concerned for her son but also appreciated that Jenny was trying to support him proactively.

Jenny thanked her and hung up. She felt a little guilty, knowing that she had not fully realised his clowning around related to his difficulty reading. She made a commitment to herself to be more sensitive to this in the future.

She also offered to provide more information to the families. They were all receptive and more than willing to provide more information themselves, particularly if it could help their child.

REFLECTION POINT

Empirical observation and data collection are transformative tools for educators, offering a systematic way to discern and understand the cues and antecedents leading to a child's behaviour. This structured methodology ensures that interventions are grounded in real patterns rather than assumptions. A truly effective support system extends beyond the classroom, and incorporating insights from parents, therapists and other caregivers creates a multidimensional perspective. By uniting in their approach, these key stakeholders deepen their collective understanding, making strategies more synchronised and effective. This collaborative endeavour bridges the gap between home, school and therapeutic environments, weaving a consistent, nurturing tapestry of caregivers for the child. A united front offers the most holistic and robust support for a child's journey.

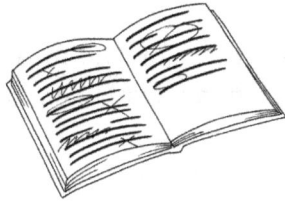

11
Decoding The Triggers

Jenny arrived at The Beach Bean before Mrs Hoo, armed with her research on her students and a warm chocolate brownie for Mrs Hoo (she had learnt about her soft spot for them from her colleagues). When Mrs Hoo arrived, she was surprised to see the brownie and green tea waiting for her. 'What's this?' she asked.

'I did my research,' Jenny replied with a cheeky grin.

'Well then,' said Mrs Hoo, impressed, 'let's get started. How did the rest of your research go?'

Jenny explained how she and Jack had been observing the kids and collecting data to identify the antecedents to their challenging behaviours. She shared the patterns they had noticed in the behaviours of Jesse, Emma and Henry.

'For instance,' Jenny said, 'when we observed Jesse during music class, free time and transitions between activities, we noticed that he often looked tense and his shoulders were raised. He also frequently had a look on his face that, at first, appeared to be a smile but wasn't. It took us a while to realise that his jaw and cheeks were tense too, and this was actually more of a tense and uncomfortable grimace than a happy smile.'

Mrs Hoo nodded thoughtfully. 'It's important to pay attention to those subtle cues,' she said. 'I am sure that information made a difference in how you responded to him.'

'It sure did,' Jenny agreed. She then went on to explain what she had identified when they observed Emma's behaviour. She had discovered that while sometimes Emma was calm and smiling prior to the event, and the hand gesture was an attempt to engage other kids, at other times she looked disorganised and unfocused and began to grind her teeth prior to the behaviour. At these times, she seemed angry or frightened and Jenny wondered if she was feeling defensive.

Mrs Hoo nodded. 'That's interesting. It shows how important it is to fully understand a child's unique profile and that there can be different reasons for the same apparent behaviour, each requiring a different strategy.'

Jenny then told Mrs Hoo about Henry's behaviour during literacy lessons, and how he would act like the class clown to avoid reading aloud. 'When we first talked about this, I sent him out of the room for disrupting the class, but then we realised, with the help of my discussion with his mother, that his behaviour was likely the result of his fear of showing he couldn't read well.'

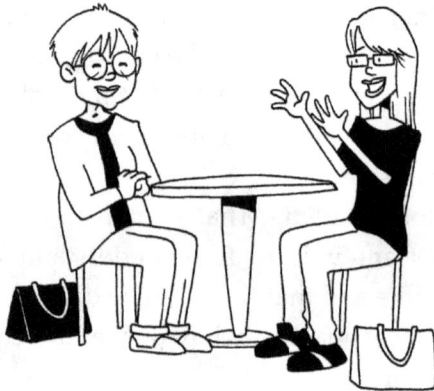

Mrs Hoo nodded. 'You're saying he didn't want to show others he had difficulty reading, so he acted in a silly way to avoid it. Is that correct?'

'Yes,' replied Jenny. 'It's almost as if he's trying to get sent out of the class or removed from the activity.'

'Because when he does,' Mrs Hoo continued, 'the consequence of his behaviour is that he avoids the reading activity, and therefore also avoids showing the class he struggles with reading.'

Jenny sat there with her mouth open. 'That's true, that is 100% what is happening.' She pondered this for a few seconds more. Still surprised at this epiphany, she said, 'Wow, back to the ABCs, huh? It's funny, I've never considered the term "consequence" in that way before. It's usually just used as a synonym for "punishment".'

Mrs Hoo nodded, her lips pressed tightly together. 'You are correct, most people think the word "consequence" means "punishment", but it actually means "whatever typically happens after the behaviour".

'This example with Henry highlights the importance of understanding the child's underlying profile and how what typically follows a behaviour can impact their response in the future.

'Today's consequence is tomorrow's antecedent,' Mrs Hoo said, summing up the concept of consequence.

'It shows how important it is to fully understand a child's unique profile and that there can be different reasons for the same apparent behaviour, each requiring a different strategy.'

REFLECTION POINT

Children's behaviours offer insights into their inner worlds and challenges. Subtle cues, like a tense smile or a seemingly defensive act, can speak volumes about a child's underlying emotions and triggers. It's imperative to observe and interpret these cues to truly understand the motives behind the child's actions. The term 'consequence' often bears a negative connotation, synonymous with 'punishment'; however, in its essence, it encompasses what naturally follows a behaviour. This understanding reshapes our approach towards consequences. As educators, health professionals and caregivers, do we recognise the broader implications of our reactions? Could we be inadvertently reinforcing behaviours we aim to deter? It's crucial to continuously evaluate our perceptions and responses so we can foster an environment where every child feels understood and supported.

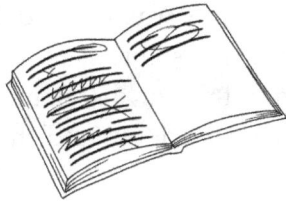

12
Consequence

Jenny repeated the phrase 'Today's consequence is tomorrow's antecedent', allowing it to sink in. 'So, you mean that what happens after the behaviour can make the behaviour more likely to occur?'

Mrs Hoo nodded and sat silently for a few seconds, letting Jenny process the idea. Then she answered, 'That's right – by understanding the child's under-lying profile and how consequences can impact behaviour, we're better equipped to support our students and help them succeed.'

Jenny was stunned. It seemed ridiculous and yet it made absolute sense. As she sat back in her chair, her mind raced, absorbing what Mrs Hoo had explained. It seemed outlandish to propose the punishment could be making the behaviour more likely, and yet it was now so obvious. The thought filled her both with trepidation and exhilarating anticipation. After what seemed like an eternity, she asked, just to make sure, 'You mean that by sending Henry out of the class or removing him from the activity, I am reinforcing the behaviour?'

'That is what I mean,' replied Mrs Hoo. 'However, there is a caveat. Having this information doesn't mean that you can continue to do this activity and simply not send him out. He still struggles with reading and feels self-conscious about it.'

'That's true,' Jenny said, thinking out loud. 'Maybe that activity isn't the best fit. Reading in front of the full group is probably quite daunting for a lot of the kids. I could stick to the smaller groups, although they can be a bit tricky for him too. What do you think?'

'I think that's a start. Perhaps you should speak to Henry, let him know that you realised requiring him to read in front of the class was a bit unfair and you're not going to do it anymore. Maybe see if he has some ideas about what might feel OK to him. You could also make sure you are giving him reading that both feels achievable and is interesting to him.'

Jenny smiled. 'OK, I can do that. Wow, once again you've shared a mountain of insights. I now see that by understanding the antecedents and consequences of their behaviour, we're better equipped to support our students and help them succeed. Any homework this week?'

'Only to continue to think about this concept. You seem to have a handle on looking at behaviours objectively, and you have done a great job at identifying the antecedents. Today we gave you a new way to look at consequence. Why don't you share this information with Jack, and continue to think about it throughout the week.'

Mrs Hoo looked at her watch. 'Oh, I need to be off. I am going out to the movies with my husband tonight, and the consequence of being late is that I will never hear the end of it.'

Jenny laughed, surprised by the joke and by the thought of a Mr Hoo. She thanked Mrs Hoo for her time and knowledge, and they headed their separate ways. Jenny realised they hadn't booked another meeting time. *Oh well*, she thought, *I feel like I have plenty to work on and to think about.* Jenny walked to her car, feeling more confident than ever about her ability to make a positive impact on her students' lives.

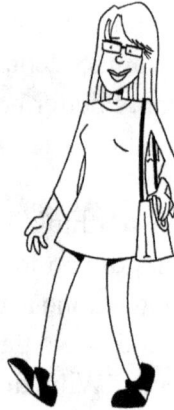

'Today's consequence is tomorrow's antecedent.'

REFLECTION POINT

Consequences are often misunderstood as punishments, but, in reality, they encompass everything that typically happens after a behaviour. Understanding the power of consequences is crucial to supporting our students effectively. It is important to consider how consequences can shape their behaviour. By recognising the impact of consequences, we can make informed decisions to provide appropriate support, and create an environment that fosters success. Reflecting on the concept of consequences helps us become more mindful of our actions and responses and their influence on the behaviours we observe in children. The consequence at the end of one chapter of a child's story sets the stage for the opening of the next chapter.

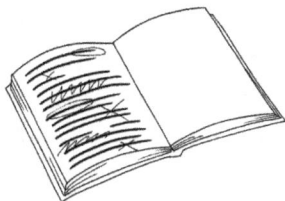

13
A Meaningful Solution

Jenny knew that the real test would be putting her new knowledge into practice with her students, especially with Henry. The next day, she decided to have a one-on-one conversation with Henry during recess. She wanted to apologise to him for sending him out of class and for making him feel uncomfortable. She also wanted to find a way to help him feel more comfortable with reading aloud in class.

'Hi, Henry,' Jenny said, approaching him on the playground. 'Do you have a moment to chat?'

Henry nodded and looked up at her with his big brown eyes. He seemed a bit nervous, but also curious.

Jenny came down to his level. 'Listen, Henry,' she began, taking a deep breath. 'I wanted to say sorry for the other day when I sent you out of class. I realise now that I wasn't being fair to you. It must have been uncomfortable for you to read in front of everyone, and I didn't consider that.'

Henry looked at her, surprised. 'It's OK, Miss. I understand,' he said softly.

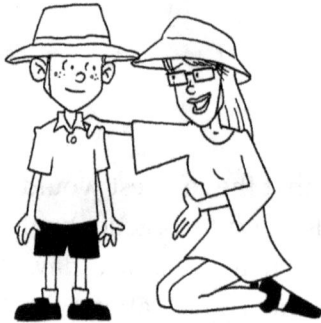

Jenny felt a wave of emotion wash over her. This little boy was so gracious and understanding, despite her mistake. She felt a pang of guilt that adults, including herself, didn't always treat children with the kindness and compassion they deserved.

'Thank you, Henry. That means a lot to me,' she said, feeling a tear form in the corner of her eye. 'So, I was thinking,' Jenny continued, wiping away the tear, 'maybe we could find a way for you to feel more comfortable reading in class. I know you like *Minecraft*, right?'

Henry's face lit up with excitement. 'Yeah, I love *Minecraft*!'

'Well, I was thinking that maybe we could get some *Minecraft* readers for the class, and you could borrow them to practise reading at home. Then, if you felt comfortable, you could read a *Minecraft* book out loud to your reading group. How does that sound?'

Henry's eyes widened. 'Really? That would be awesome!'

Jenny smiled. She felt relieved that Henry was so receptive to her suggestion. This was exactly the kind of meaningful, relevant and motivating activity she had learnt about in her conversation with Mrs Hoo. She also felt proud of herself for repairing her relationship with Henry and building trust with him.

Over the next couple of weeks, Jenny worked with Henry to find *Minecraft* readers that were at his reading level. She also made sure to check in with him regularly to see how he was doing with his reading practice. Henry was motivated and engaged now that he was reading a book that was meaningful to him, and he seemed to be enjoying the process.

Then, one day in class, Henry raised his hand during reading time. Jenny called on him and he stood up nervously. He had a *Minecraft* book in his hands.

'Miss, can I read this out loud to the class?' he asked.

Jenny's heart swelled with pride. She knew that this was a big step for Henry. 'Of course, Henry. I'd love for you to share your reading with the class.'

Henry took a deep breath and began to read. His voice was shaky at first, but then it became stronger and more confident. The other kids in the class listened attentively, and when he finished they clapped and cheered.

Jenny felt a tear roll down her cheek. She knew that this moment was about so much more than just reading a book. It was about building relationships, repairing trust and showing children they were valued and respected.

As the class settled down, Jenny looked at Henry and smiled. 'Great job, Henry. You read wonderfully.'

Henry beamed with pride.

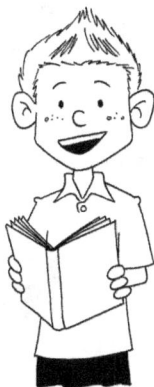

*She knew that this moment was about so much
more than just reading a book. It was about
building relationships, repairing trust and showing
children they were valued and respected.*

REFLECTION POINT

Jenny and Henry's interactions about finding motivating
readers for Henry demonstrates the transformative power
of meaningful relationships and leveraging children's
interests in the learning process. When we take the time
to build genuine connections and tap into what truly
engages our children, remarkable transformations occur.
By recognising and embracing their individual interests,
such as Henry's love for *Minecraft*, educators can create

meaningful and relevant learning experiences that motivate and empower students. This serves as a reminder of the immense impact that personalisation, compassion and nurturing relationships can have on students' educational journeys, fostering their growth, confidence and love for learning.

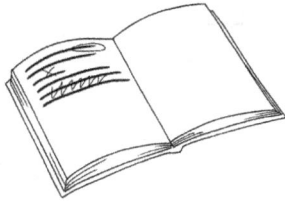

14
Parent–Teacher Interviews

Jenny sat behind her desk in her classroom with her laptop, surrounded by a pile of folders. It was parent–teacher interview day, and one by one parents were coming in to discuss their child's progress. She had a wonderful conversation with Emma's father about how Emma was now successfully joining in a lot more activities. She also spoke to Jesse's mother. Jesse had made some great gains too, although he was still struggling socially, particularly on the playground. Next up were Henry's parents. Jenny was particularly looking forward to this conversation, as Henry was improving significantly in both reading and behaviour.

Henry's parents entered the classroom, looking a bit wary and nervous. They had received positive feedback from Jenny in the past, but they were still hesitant to get their hopes up.

'Hello, it's great to see you both. Please, take a seat,' she said, gesturing towards the chairs in front of her desk.

Henry's mother sat down and began, 'We've been looking forward to this meeting. It's been a long time since we've received any positive feedback about Henry's progress at school, so we're a bit nervous.'

Jenny could sense the trepidation in her voice, and immediately responded with a reassuring smile. 'I understand, but I think you'll be pleasantly surprised by what I have to say.'

Henry's mother nodded, and Jenny told them about how Henry had been doing in class, sharing examples of his progress and successes. As she spoke, she could see the relief on their faces.

Henry's mother then mentioned they had started to get him some therapy. 'His speech therapist said even though he is fine at talking, he has some difficulty processing certain sounds. Apparently, that can also make reading hard. She referred us to an occupational therapist, who thinks he has some visual perceptual issues, which they are working on.'

Jenny listened carefully and reflected on Henry's underlying differences, which were making it hard for him to read but weren't obvious to the eye. She made a mental note about how important it was to know about the child's abilities and challenges when looking at behaviour.

'I see,' Jenny said, nodding thoughtfully. 'It's good he's getting the support he needs. It's important to understand the whole picture when it comes to learning difficulties. I've actually been using some new techniques in the classroom that seem to be helping Henry.'

Henry's mother leaned forward, eager to hear more.

Jenny continued, 'I've been working on finding activities and materials that are interesting to him, and I've also been giving him choices. For example, I bought the *Minecraft* readers with him in mind.'

Henry's mother's eyes widened. 'Wow, I was surprised when he brought them home, but in a happy way. I'd never seen him so willing to do homework.

What's more surprising is that he has asked if we can buy some more. He's asking to buy books. It's unbelievable!' She paused, as if to swallow a sob. 'Thank you for taking the time to find something that works for him.'

Jenny smiled. 'It's my pleasure. I'm just happy to see him enjoying school and making such great progress.'

As the meeting was winding down, Jenny became aware of the profound silence from Henry's father. He had sat quietly throughout, his face carrying a mix of expressions – thoughtful, guarded and hopeful. It was clear he was deeply invested in his son's progress, even if he chose not to express this verbally. She had observed this quiet strength in Henry too, yet she couldn't help but feel uneasy, wondering what he was thinking. Her fears were quickly relieved. As Henry's parents were gathering their things to leave, his father finally spoke: 'I just wanted to say I appreciate everything you've done for Henry. It means a lot to us that you see the good in him,' he said with a nod, before following his wife out the door.

Jenny was touched by his words and couldn't help but feel a sense of pride in the progress Henry had made. As his parents left the room, she thought about how far he had come and how much further he could go with the right support.

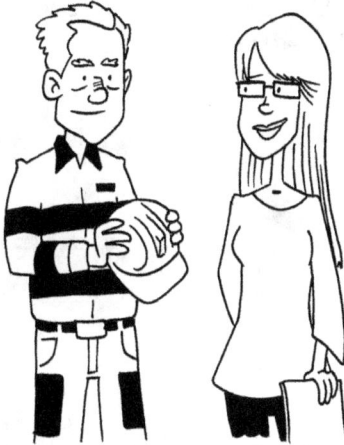

She made a mental note about how important it was to know about the child's abilities and challenges when looking at behaviour.

REFLECTION POINT

The power of seeing the good in every child and fostering unconditional positive regard is transformative. By recognising and building on their strengths, adults can inspire confidence and facilitate remarkable growth in their students. A team approach can be powerful, and that team can include parents, teachers, therapists and the child. By working collaboratively, the child's support team can help the child to progress on their own hero's journey, moving through the struggle to victory.

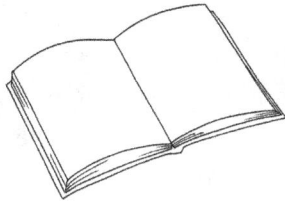

15
The Playground

The next day, Jenny felt unshakable. Her students were kicking goals left, right and centre, and the night before, she had shared all those wins with their parents. As she was finishing her lunch, however, Bill Roberts, a veteran of the school's faculty, strode towards Jenny. Bill's teaching style, formed over years of experience, was as straight and unbending as his posture. With a perpetually furrowed brow and stern voice, he ruled his classroom with an iron fist and had little patience for students who stepped out of line. His reputation for strict discipline was known throughout the school, and even Jenny, despite her differing teaching philosophy, couldn't help but feel a twinge of anxiety when he approached with an angry look on his face.

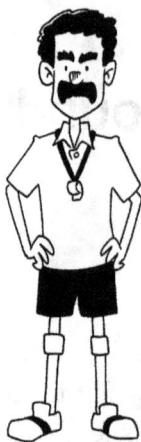

'You need to do something about that Jesse Thompson kid. He's started a fight again at lunch. Biffed Ethan Nyugen from my class. We'll have his mother up here for sure.' Jesse, despite making strides in the classroom, had a long-standing record of having issues with his peers on the playground, leaving the children in tears and the teachers at their wits' end.

'What happened?' Jenny asked, trying to keep her cool. Bill had a way of making her hold her breath.

'I told you what happened. He biffed him! What more do you need to know?' he responded.

'What I mean is...' Jenny drew up all her courage. 'What I mean is, why did it happen? Behaviours don't happen in a vacuum. There's always a context, with an antecedent and a consequence.'

'I'll tell you why. 'Cos he's a thug. What happened before it? Nothing. What's the consequence? The consequence is that now I have to go tell the other kid's mother, and she's not gonna be happy. I don't have time for this,' he huffed. 'I have to go call Kim Nyugen. Just sort him out.' He stormed off.

Jenny sat back down, staring at her sandwich. She knew that Jesse was struggling, and she had been working hard to support him. In class he was doing well, but he was still having a lot of difficulty at lunchtimes and she just couldn't be there every minute of the day to help him. She felt helpless, not knowing what to do next. She couldn't help but wonder what antecedent led to the behaviour, and what it was in his profile that made him so susceptible to reacting this way.

She finished her lunch, feeling uneasy, and wondered how she was going to approach the situation with Jesse and Bill.

She couldn't help but wonder what antecedent led to the behaviour, and what it was in his profile that made him so susceptible to reacting this way.

REFLECTION POINT

It's important to understand the context and underlying causes of a child's behaviour, even in challenging situations. Behaviours do not occur in isolation, but are influenced by antecedents and consequences. By seeking to understand and address the underlying factors, we can approach behaviour with empathy and find effective solutions that support positive outcomes for all involved.

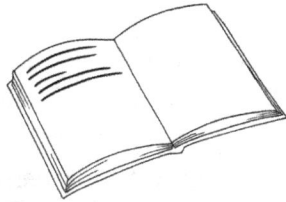

16

Behaviour Management Plan

The next day Jenny and Mrs Hoo had a break from their classes at the same time. Mrs Hoo was marking some assignments and Jenny sat down next to her. 'Hi, Mrs Hoo, have you got a minute?'

Mrs Hoo put down her pen and turned her whole body towards Jenny. 'Of course, Jenny, how have you been?'

'Overall, pretty good,' Jenny answered. 'I've learnt so much from you this term about how to help my students with their behaviours. I know to always start by being objective, looking at how the child appeared when an incident happened and thinking about why it might have happened. I also look at what happens afterwards to see if that could be contributing to future behaviours. Oh, and I've realised how important it is that I consider their individual differences too.'

Mrs Hoo listened intently, nodding at each point Jenny mentioned.

Jenny continued, 'I've been thinking, though, that's all well and good when I'm there to support them or when I see it happening; but I'm not always there and I can't be there all the time.'

'Hmm, that is true—' said Mrs Hoo.

'For instance,' Jenny interrupted, anxious to get Mrs Hoo's help, 'I know that every day when Jesse goes out on that playground he's going to end up hitting someone.'

'Well,' said Mrs Hoo, eyebrows raised, 'maybe you need a behaviour management plan.'

'We've tried those,' Jenny responded, almost without thought, 'but there's nothing we can put in them that seems to stop him from getting into fights.'

'Sorry, I think you misunderstood me,' replied Mrs Hoo. 'If you know there's going to be a fight or a child's going to hit another child and you leave it up to them, then maybe *you* need a behaviour management plan... for yourself.

'He's only six years old, Jenny. Kids don't have great executive functions or the ability to understand consequences until they are older. Actually, that skill isn't fully developed until twenty-five. Don't get me wrong, many kids can do this, but it is still developing. If the child's regulation is challenged, either because they're upset or overexcited, then they won't have access to this at all.'

She let that sink in for a few seconds. Then she added, 'They might not have access to their thinking and reasoning brain, Jenny, but I'm hoping you do. Let's think about how you, and the other adults, could help. Have you noticed any bright spots? Any times when he managed to avoid a fight, maybe with the help of an adult?'

'Well actually, yes, I have,' Jenny answered. 'Just last week when I was on playground duty, he came up and said hi to me at the start of lunch. I remember crouching down and saying hello to him. I also said, "Now Jesse, remember, there's no fighting, OK? If you need my help, I'm right here. Got it?" He nodded and said "Yes, Miss Jones," and then he ran off to play. Then, would you believe it? When he had a disagreement with one of his peers, he came and found me, and I helped them work it out. But I can't be there all the time,' she finished.

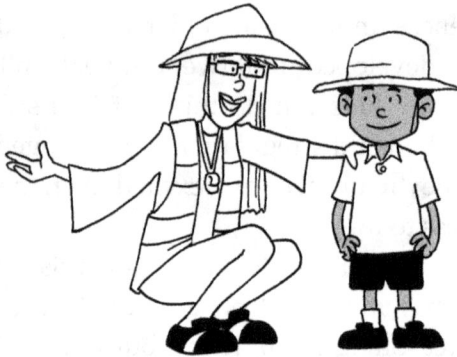

Mrs Hoo looked at Jenny. She had come so far. 'You are becoming skilled at supporting kids, but was it that you have some magical aura and this could only be done by you? Or was it that you connected with him, and, in doing so, gave him an anchor, an ally, a reference point for support? Then you rehearsed a strategy, close to the time he needed it, so that when his regulation was challenged he had a strategy close to mind and could use the support of a trusted ally and avoid getting into a fight.'

This was a lot to take in. Jenny listened and felt she was starting to understand. It felt like one of those *Magic Eye* puzzles: she could see there was something there, but she couldn't quite conceive what the answer was.

'They might not have access to their thinking and reasoning brain, Jenny, but I'm hoping you do.'

REFLECTION POINT

Being proactive is often more effective than being reactive, whether in the classroom, the clinic or at home. Prevention is always better than intervention. Educators, health professionals and parents/caregivers have the power to shape environments and situations in ways that set children up for success. By foreseeing potential challenges and equipping children with strategies ahead of time, we can create a nurturing environment where they feel supported and understood. It's an encouragement for all stakeholders in a child's life to think deeply, adapt and be willing to view challenges from a different perspective.

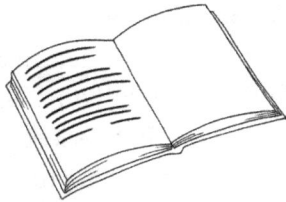

17

Empowering With Responsibility

'You're not there every lunchtime, but someone is, right? Are they easy to find?' Mrs Hoo asked, already knowing the answer.

'They're wearing a bright yellow vest, so I'd say so,' replied Jenny, the image of the solution starting to take shape.

'Even so,' Mrs Hoo continued, 'that might not be so easy when Jesse's regulation is challenged, and he has to think about finding them. What if he could be in charge of giving something to the teacher on duty?

A note or an object, like a whistle or a ball? When he hands it to the teacher, they could get down to his level, just like you did, connect eye to eye with him and say, "Hey Jesse, thank you for being so responsible and delivering me this note. If you need anything or have a tricky time with your friends, just look for my yellow vest and come find me, and I'll help you work it out." This will give him a reference point and an ally. It will also help him quickly rehearse a plan, just like you did. It will allow the teacher to watch where he goes to play so they can keep an eye and ear out. If it gets a little rowdy, they can pop over before it gets out of hand and coach the kids through it.'

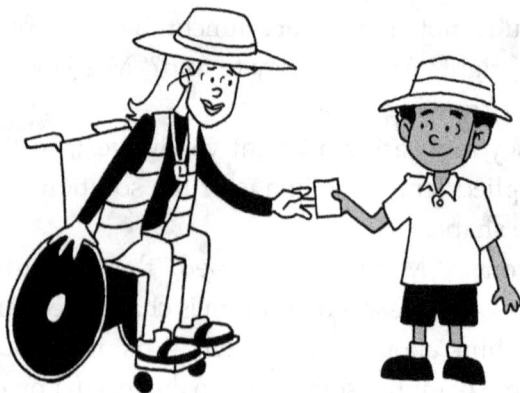

Jenny felt a sense of relief and gratitude as Mrs Hoo's words sank in. She realised that it wasn't about finding a perfect solution or trying to control every moment of the day, but providing support and resources for the child to use in the moment. She felt empowered by the idea of giving Jesse the responsibility of delivering something 'important' to the teacher on duty, and providing him with a trusted ally on the playground, someone he could turn to when he needed help.

As she walked back to her classroom, Jenny couldn't help but think about the progress she had made in her approach to behaviour management. She felt grateful for the guidance and support of Mrs Hoo and for the opportunity to learn and grow alongside her students. She also knew that there were still challenges ahead and there was always room for improvement. She made a mental note to continue reflecting on her practice and to seek out resources and support whenever she needed them.

As she entered her classroom, Jenny felt a renewed sense of purpose and excitement for the work ahead. She knew that it wouldn't be easy, but she was ready to face whatever challenges came her way and felt committed to learning and growing alongside her students. The next challenge was figuring out how to get the school and staff on board with supporting Jesse at lunchtimes.

> *'This will give him a reference point and an ally. It will also help him quickly rehearse a plan, just like you did.'*

REFLECTION POINT

Empowering children with proactive behaviour management plans allows them to take responsibility and actively seek out support when faced with challenges. Adults, be it teachers, therapists, parents or caregivers, play an essential role in offering this guidance. By connecting with students and providing clear strategies, adults can foster trust, strengthen relationships and create an environment conducive to learning. This approach helps children develop self-regulation skills and fosters a sense of responsibility and agency in their behaviour choices. It provides them with tools to write their new story, make positive choices and face adversities with confidence.

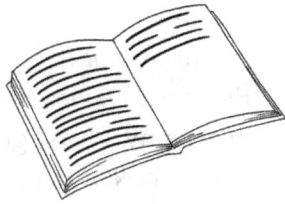

18
Staff Meeting

Jenny walked into the staffroom, clutching a folder that contained her proposal for a new approach to behaviour management. She took a seat among her colleagues, feeling a mix of nervousness and determination.

As the meeting began, Principal Davies addressed the staff, discussing various school matters. When there was a lull in the conversation, Jenny seized the opportunity to speak up. 'Excuse me, Principal Davies, may I share an idea I have for supporting one of my students?' Her voice was steady, despite the slight tremor in her hands.

Principal Davies nodded with a warm smile. 'Of course, Jenny. Please go ahead.'

Jenny took a deep breath and began to explain her observations on Jesse's behaviour and her proposed plan for providing him with support on the playground. She outlined the idea of giving him a responsibility and connecting him with the teacher on playground duty.

As she finished, she looked around the room to gauge her colleagues' reactions. Most appeared thoughtful, but Bill Roberts, sitting across the table, scoffed loudly and interjected, 'Are you serious, Jenny? Giving special treatment to a troublemaker? That won't solve anything.' His tone was dripping with scepticism.

Principal Davies raised an eyebrow and cleared his throat. 'Bill, I appreciate your perspective, but let's remember that our goal here is to support all of our students, regardless of their challenges. Jenny has come up with an innovative approach that could make a significant difference for Jesse and the students he sometimes has trouble with. You know, Bill, like Ethan in your class.'

Bill crossed his arms and rolled his eyes, clearly unconvinced, but at the mention of Ethan he hesitated slightly. It was true that Ethan often found himself at odds with Jesse. It was a struggle Bill knew all too well. He let out a sigh, his sceptical expression softening just a bit as he considered Principal Davies's words.

Principal Davies continued, addressing the whole staff: 'In this school we prioritise inclusivity, empathy and finding individualised solutions for our students. Jenny's proposal aligns perfectly with these values. I think it's important we support her in implementing this plan.'

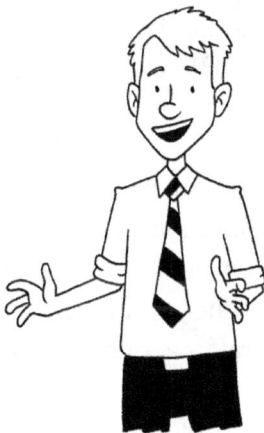

The room was quiet as Principal Davies's words resonated. Most of the teachers were attentive and nodded supportively. Jenny felt a surge of gratitude.

Principal Davies turned to her. 'Jenny, I commend your dedication and creativity. Let's schedule a meeting to discuss the details and ensure we have the necessary support in place.'

Jenny's face lit up with a mix of relief and excitement. She nodded gratefully, feeling a renewed sense of purpose and confidence. She noticed Mrs Hoo sitting quietly to her left. When they made eye contact, Mrs Hoo gave her a wink of acknowledgement and respect at Jenny's courage and passion for helping her students.

As the meeting continued, Jenny noticed a shift in the atmosphere. Her colleagues began discussing ideas and sharing their own strategies for supporting students with challenging behaviours. The staffroom became a space for collaboration and growth, with everyone recognising the importance of their collective responsibility in creating a positive and inclusive learning environment within their school.

Jenny left the staff meeting that day with a sense of pride, knowing that her voice had been heard and that she had the support of her colleagues and Principal

Davies. She was eager to implement her plan and make a positive impact on Jesse's life as well as the lives of other students facing similar challenges.

Jenny thought about the power of teamwork and collective effort in fostering an environment where every student could thrive. The staff meeting had become a turning point, marking the beginning of a collaborative journey towards better support and understanding for all students at the school.

'Let's remember that our goal here is to support all of our students, regardless of their challenges.'

REFLECTION POINT

As adults who support children, we have a collective responsibility to foster inclusive environments where every child is given the opportunity to succeed. As educators, therapists and caregivers, it is our role to create and implement individualised strategies that meet the unique needs of the children we support. These strategies should not only address children's challenges but also support them in creating a new narrative for themselves, allowing for successful participation and interactions.

Implementing a proactive approach such as the one proposed by Jenny can seem daunting, but there is tremendous benefit to fostering a collaborative environment and harnessing the power of teamwork. Sharing ideas and experiences, and collectively supporting innovative strategies, is critical in shifting the trajectory for children with challenging behaviours. By doing so, we are not only creating a supportive learning environment but also empowering children to write their new story.

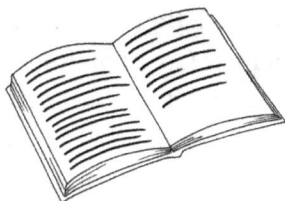

19

Goodbye, Mrs Hoo

Jenny walked down the cold, empty hallway, feeling a mix of emotions. She was excited about all she had learnt from Mrs Hoo but sad it was now time to say goodbye to her new mentor. Tom Reed was due to return on Monday, which meant that Mrs Hoo's time at Green Beach Public School had come to an end. She knew that Mrs Hoo had made a significant impact on her teaching and on the lives of her students.

As she approached Tom Reed's classroom, she took a deep breath and knocked on the door. Mrs Hoo opened the door and smiled when she saw Jenny. 'Jenny! Come on in. It's nice to see you,' she said, her eyes sparkling and warm.

Jenny handed Mrs Hoo a present. 'This is for you. A little thank you for everything you've done for me and my students.'

Mrs Hoo took the gift from Jenny – a bonsai tree. 'Jenny, this is lovely. Thank you so much. I have always thought bonsais are beautiful. What type is it?'

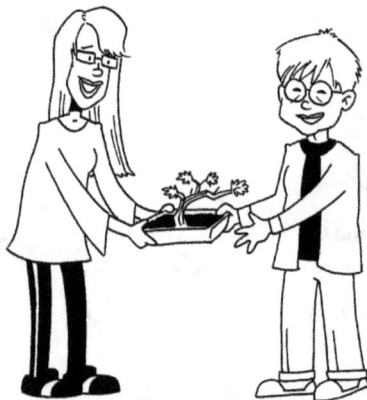

'It's a Japanese maple tree,' Jenny answered. 'It symbolises balance, harmony and practicality. I read that in Japanese culture it is also a symbol of love. Oh, and it is often associated with the idea of transformation, as the tree changes its appearance and colours throughout the seasons.'

'Once again, you have done your research.' Mrs Hoo smiled at Jenny, proud at how far she had come in such a short time and genuinely glad to have had the chance to meet this wonderful young teacher.

They both sat down, and Jenny reflected on all the transformations that had taken place in her classroom over the past few months. 'Mrs Hoo, I can't thank you enough for everything you've taught me. My students have made incredible progress and I've learnt so much about how to support them.'

Mrs Hoo smiled, nodding in agreement. 'It's been a pleasure to work with you, Jenny. I'm so proud of all the work you've done.'

Jenny accepted the compliment with a smile, and continued listing all the things she had learnt from Mrs Hoo. 'It's truly amazing how much I have gained from your mentorship. I've learnt so much about my students and their behaviour, and about the importance of looking at behaviours objectively. Looking at how the child is responding helps me move from focusing on the "what" of the behaviour to the "why". Keeping it objective takes the emotion out of it, allowing me to let the data drive my thinking. Behaviours never happen in a vacuum; there is always a context or a wider story that can be revealed.

'I now understand that identifying the antecedent can help us know what led to the behaviour, and that this might be from just before but could also be from a much earlier time. What typically happens after a behaviour, the consequence, can also impact the likelihood of the behaviour happening again. A wise woman once said "Today's consequence is tomorrow's antecedent".' Mrs Hoo accepted the compliment with a raise of her eyebrows.

'I've also learnt,' Jenny continued, 'about how the child's underlying capacities and challenges can impact their ability to learn, engage and regulate their emotions. I've discovered the power of working collaboratively with the child and incorporating their ideas and interests, the things that are meaningful and motivating to them.

'In my search to better understand the context, I've learnt important lessons on the importance of taking responsibility as adults who have working executive functions (hopefully) and the value of collaborating as a team. Although, I sometimes question whether those executive functions are always fully developed in adults, especially when I'm talking to Bill Roberts. He's got a few regulation challenges, I think.'

Mrs Hoo gave a chuckle. 'You're right, it's hard for kids, and sometimes even adults, to access their thinking, reasoning and language when regulation is challenged. It's important for us adults to have an active role in helping students develop these skills.'

Jenny smiled. 'Yes, that's right! At those times, they don't have access to their thinking brains, but hopefully we adults do.

'I know that I have so much more to learn,' Jenny continued, 'and I'm excited to continue to grow and to support my students to grow. I even found myself sharing this advice with Casey in 1C. She has some similar kids in her class.'

Mrs Hoo smiled back. 'I have no doubt that you will continue to make a positive impact in your students' lives for a long time, and also in the lives of your colleagues and future mentees.'

As they said their goodbyes, Jenny felt a deep sense of gratitude for everything Mrs Hoo had taught her. She knew that her students had been changed for the better because of Mrs Hoo's guidance, and she would always be thankful for that.

As she walked out of the classroom, Jenny knew that she was ready to continue her journey as a teacher, armed with new knowledge and skills. Even though Mrs Hoo would not be there in person, Jenny would always carry her lessons and spirit with her.

'I'm excited to continue to grow and to support my students to grow. I even found myself sharing this advice with Casey in 1C. She has some similar kids in her class.'

REFLECTION POINT

As educators, therapists, parents and caregivers, we are always learning and growing. We can never know everything, so it's important to seek out support. It's also important for workplaces and our communities to provide support to the families who support their children.

There is an African proverb that says 'It takes a village to raise a child'. At times, we can feel isolated and alone in our quest. This quote should serve as a reminder that we cannot do it alone. As an extension, we should not put this expectation on others. As businesses, community networks, friends and colleagues, we need to support the people who support the kids. As individuals, the most courageous and caring thing we can do for the children we support is to ask for support when we need it to help us help the child.

It's important to allow ourselves to be learners, and to consolidate that learning by sharing it with others.

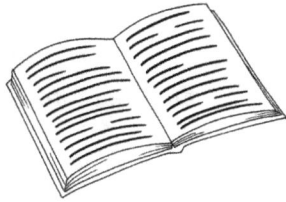

Epilogue:
The Wise Old Owl

As Jenny headed for her car, she walked past a group of children playing 'magic wand' as they waited for their bus. She stopped for a minute to soak in their joy and watch their game unfold.

'Abracadabra, now you're all dogs,' the little girl said as the others began to crawl and woof. She raised her magic wand again and said, 'Abracadabra, now you're all owls.'

'Hoo, hoo, hoo,' they all began, waving their arms and soaring through the sky.

'Hoo!' Jenny exclaimed, joining in with the children's game. Her unexpected participation brought giggles and delighted glances from the kids.

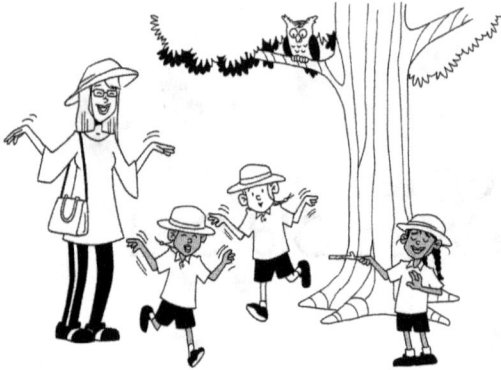

While the wise old owl's time at Green Beach Public School had come to an end, she knew that her influence would continue to resonate with Jenny, and, subsequently, with all the students Jenny would teach in the future.

When you connect with someone, you become a part of their story. When you help them grow, you help them create a new narrative. They now hold the pen to their own story, and the possibility of a happy ending is within reach.

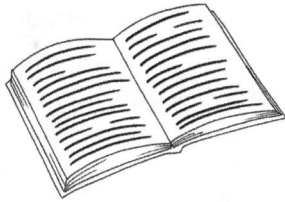

Conclusion

This story is a testament to all the amazing people supporting children with behaviours we find challenging. Through Jenny's experiences and the guidance of Mrs Hoo, we see the transformative power of empathy, understanding and collaborative effort. This journey into the heart of behavioural understanding emphasises the importance of viewing children's actions not just as mere behaviours but as a language – a manifestation of their underlying capacities, experiences and environment.

Jenny's story highlights the importance of treating each child as a unique individual. In doing so, it underscores both the value of viewing behaviours objectively, identifying antecedents and consequences, and the indispensability of working hand in hand with a child's primary support structures, especially parents and caregivers.

The story also provides a deeper layer in illustrating the relationship of support and growth between Jenny and Mrs Hoo. This relationship embodies the principle of 'supporting the people who support the kids'. It encapsulates a message not only for teachers but also for healthcare professionals, parents, caregivers and anyone involved in the process of nurturing a young mind. The story emphasises that for children to truly rewrite their narratives, there must be a concerted effort from all their guiding lights – teachers, families and the community at large.

Transcending the pages of the story, MoveAbout also seeks to embody this principle, which serves as a beacon for everyone involved in a child's developmental journey. This is not merely a tag line but serves as the heart of every initiative and decision made within the MoveAbout framework. This support extends, without boundaries, to families, MoveAbout team members and the broader community.

Through the MoveAbout Learning Pathways courses, the one-on-one MoveAbout Mentoring or the MoveAbout Immersion Program, the MoveAbout team seek to provide a platform for occupational therapists and others to grow and learn with support. The team reinforce this narrative's message of connection, collaboration, lifelong learning and hands-on experience. The programs are channels that bridge theory and practice, creating an environment that is as much about understanding children as it is about empowering those who support them.

I hope that you have enjoyed this story and the lessons within. I also hope that you have begun to consider your own story moving forward and how you will use this knowledge to support both kids and the people who support kids in your life.

Beyond our clinics, MoveAbout also supports our community through our MoveAbout Learning Pathways courses, MoveAbout Mentoring and MoveAbout Immersion Programs.

MoveAbout Learning Pathways

MoveAbout Learning Pathways is dedicated to the enrichment and support of professionals and caregivers supporting children. We offer a blend of innovative workshops and courses, including in-person sessions led by renowned figures in occupational therapy, such as Julia Wilbarger and Kim Barthel, as well as MoveAbout original content. With a foundational belief in the power of ongoing education and connection, MoveAbout embodies the values of lifelong learning and purposeful impact. Whether it's through our engaging live workshops or online content, our mission is clear: to support the people who support the kids.

Find out more at: www.moveabout.com.au/ courses.

MoveAbout Mentoring Program

The MoveAbout Mentoring Program is designed for paediatric occupational therapists to receive regular clinical and professional mentoring to support them in their work with kids and families. The program includes a MoveAbout Mentoring Scholarship for therapists who are not receiving adequate supervision or mentoring at their current workplace. Sessions are conducted via Zoom or in person at a MoveAbout clinic on a weekly, fortnightly or monthly basis.

Find out more at: www.moveabout.com.au/courses.

MoveAbout Immersion Program

The MoveAbout Immersion Program is a five-day immersion experience that provides a rare opportunity to dive into the methods and culture of the MoveAbout Therapy Services clinics. The program includes a comprehensive overview of the Move-About approach to paediatric occupational therapy, including the client journey, systems, equipment, tools and resources we use to support clinical reasoning and treatment. Participants have the opportunity to observe and participate in occupational therapy sessions. They also receive daily one-on-one educational meetings with members of our team. The program is tailored to the individual needs and interests of each participant, and will provide an invaluable experience for those interested in expand-ing and developing their knowledge of paediatric occupational therapy.

Find out more at: www.moveabout.com.au/courses.

Acknowledgements

From the beginning of this journey, as I tapped notes into my phone with the Western Australian Desert rolling by and Kathy at the wheel, the steady support of my wife and our children, Harry and Hugo, was palpable. Their constant encouragement, love and understanding – even when I was late for dinner – became the bedrock of my resilience throughout the arduous writing process. I must emphasise that any idea or insight I present is intrinsically tied to

Kathy – an exceptional occupational therapist and an even more remarkable mother and wife.

Gratitude is also due to my mum; my sisters, Maree and Gen; my stepfather, Peter; and the extended clan of uncles, aunties and cousins: we are a lineage of nurturers – teachers, principals, librarians, social workers, occupational therapists and disability support workers. This vibrant tapestry of caregivers has been the origin of my creative and compassionate spirit.

To the diligent MoveAbout team: your unwavering commitment, infectious enthusiasm and shared vision have been the foundation of this endeavour. Your ceaseless efforts transcend this book, breathing life into our mission and ensuring it creates a lasting impact. Here's to a world where all kids, regardless of their differences, can live meaningful lives and be valued and valuable members of their communities.

In my professional voyage, I have been fortunate to have mentors who've served as guiding stars. Their invaluable insights are woven into every page of this book. Thank you to Colleen Hacker for the empowering mantra 'This is hard and you can do it!' This is a phrase I have used to support every child and family, and also a phrase that has motivated and anchored me during challenging times – and possibly gotten me to the end of this book. To Beth Osten, my first employer and mentor in paediatric occupational therapy (OT), for guiding me as I discovered the Developmental, Individual-difference, Relationship-based model. This has reshaped my outlook, placing the child – not their behaviour – at the core of our support. You instilled in me a high standard for supporting the people who support the kids through supervision, in-session coaching and professional development. To Tracy Stackhouse, for your enlightening introduction to the STEPPSI model and the ABC-Iceberg, which have both made my professional compass more accurate and expanded and deepened my clinical reasoning in regard to children and behaviour.

A special note of gratitude to other mentors who have been pivotal in my journey and the growth of the MoveAbout team: Sheila Frick, Kim Barthel, Sherri Cawn, Gil Foley, Julia Wilbarger, Patricia Wilbarger, Mary Kawar and Patti Oetter. Your wisdom, mentorship and generous hearts have been indispensable. To all I've named and those I haven't yet whose influence has been just as profound, I offer my deepest thanks. Your collective spirit and contributions have given rise to this book and enhanced our shared experience. With deepest appreciation, Dave.

The Author

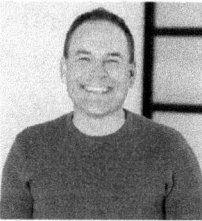

Dave Jereb is a visionary paediatric occupational therapist who has shown unwavering commitment to enhancing the lives of children for over two decades. Dave and his equally dedicated wife, Kathy, co-founded MoveAbout Therapy Services in 2008 and have revolutionised paediatric occupational therapy in Australia. Central to Dave's philosophy is the belief 'We support the people who support the kids'.

Dave passionately advocates the best way to assist children is by empowering the adults in their lives – parents, caregivers, allied health professionals and educators – with the tools to read, understand and positively influence their behaviour. This core principle is evident in MoveAbout's promise to offer unparalleled therapy and support, ensuring that children, regardless of their differences, have the opportunity to lead meaningful lives and become valued and valuable members of their communities.

A staunch advocate for continuous learning and development, Dave, in collaboration with Kathy, crafted the MoveAbout Activity Cards and developed transformative workshops, including 'A Dynamic Approach to Regulation and Behaviour' and 'Connecting with Kids with ASD'. Dave's contributions also include co-presenting the online course 'STEPPSI: A Tool For Effective Clinical Reasoning' with Tracy Stackhouse, and the in-person live course 'Sensory Defensiveness: A Comprehensive Treatment Approach' alongside Dr Julia Wilbarger.

Beyond the bounds of MoveAbout, Dave has been a guiding star to early career OTs and the businesses who employ them, battling burnout and striving to nurture their professional growth. As a mentor and coach, he's passionate about uplifting the community, fostering connections and injecting a playful spirit into the process of lifelong learning. His expertise shines through multiple platforms, from podcasts like *Chatabout Children with Sonia Bestulic*, *Private Practice Made Perfect with Cathy Love*, *Run Like Clockwork* and *Holly the OT Podcast* to enriching series on the MoveAbout Therapy Services YouTube channel, such as *Beach Topics* and *MoveAbout Supervision Sessions*.

In every endeavour, Dave brings along his relentless dedication, keen insights and an unwavering spirit of service. With his vast experience and a heart anchored in making a difference, he is undeniably shaping a brighter future for paediatric OT in Australia.

⊕ www.moveabout.com.au

🅵 www.facebook.com/MoveAboutTherapy

🅻 www.linkedin.com/in/dave-jereb-039b2a4/

🅾 http://www.instagram.com/davejereb_ot/

🅾 http://www.instagram.com/moveabout.ot/

▶ www.youtube.com/@
MoveAboutTherapyServices